Slow Cooker

Illustrated Paleo Crock Pot Recipes With Delicious Slow Cooker Soups, Stews, Dinners, Sides And Desserts

(The Complete Slow Cooker Recipe)

Kirk Simon

Table Of Contents

Artichoke And Spinach Dip

Ingredients:

- 1 cup 2% milk
- 2 package cream cheese, at room temperature
- 2 cup grated Parmesan cheese
- 1/2 teaspoon sea salt
- ⅛ teaspoon freshly ground black pepper
- 2 can artichoke hearts, drained and chopped
- 2 cups frozen chopped spinach, thawed and squeezed dry
- 2 tablespoon minced garlic

Directions

1. Place the artichoke hearts, spinach, garlic, milk, cream cheese, Parmesan, salt, and pepper in a 2-quart slow cooker.

2. Stir well to combine.

3. Cover and cook on low for 2 hours, or until the cheese is melted and the dip is hot.

4. Serve the dip in the slow cooker with the heat on low or "keep warm."

Mushroom Dip

Ingredients:

- 2 garlic cloves, minced
- A pinch of salt and black pepper
- 2 tablespoon balsamic vinegar
- 1 tablespoon basil, chopped
- 1 tablespoon oregano, chopped
- 4 ounces white mushrooms, chopped
- 2 eggplant, cubed
- 1 cup heavy cream
- 1 tablespoon tahini paste

Directions:

1. In your slow cooker, mix the mushrooms with the fresh egg plant, cream, and the other ingredients, toss, put the lid on and cook on High for 6 hours.

2. Divide the mushroom mix into bowls and serve as a dip.

Raspberry Chia Pudding

Ingredients:

- 2 cup of coconut milk

- 2 teaspoons raspberries

- 4 tablespoons chia seeds

Directions:

1. Put chia seeds and coconut milk in the Slow Cooker and cook it for 2 hours on Low.

2. Then transfer the cooked chia pudding to the glasses and top with raspberries.

Ham Omelet

Ingredients:

- 2 small yellow onion, chopped
- 1 cup ham, chopped
- 1 cup cheddar cheese, shredded
- 2 tablespoon chives, chopped
- A pinch of salt and black pepper
- Cooking spray
- 4 eggs, whisked
- 2 tablespoon sour cream
- 2 spring onions, chopped

Directions:

1. Grease your Slow Cooker with the cooking spray and mix the eggs with the sour cream, spring onions, and the other ingredients inside.

2. Toss the mix, spread into the pot, put the lid on, and cook on High for 4 hours.

3. Divide the mix between plates and serve for breakfast right away.

Crab Dip

Ingredients:

- 2 garlic cloves, minced
- Juice of 2 lemon
- 2   and 1 tablespoon Worcestershire sauce
- 2 and 1 teaspoons old bay seasoning
- 1 ounces crabmeat
- 1 ounces cream cheese
- 1 cup parmesan, grated
- 1 cup mayonnaise
- 1 cup green onions, chopped

Directions:

1. In your slow cooker, mix cream cheese with parmesan, mayo, green onions, garlic, lemon juice, Worcestershire sauce, old bay seasoning, and crabmeat, stir, cover, and cook on Low for 2 hours.

2. Divide into bowls and serve as a dip.

Chickpeas Spread

Ingredients:

- 2 tablespoon tahini
- A pinch of salt and black pepper
- 2 garlic clove, minced
- 1 tablespoon chives, chopped
- 1 cup chickpeas, dried
- 2 tablespoon olive oil
- 2 tablespoon lemon juice
- 2 cup veggie stock

Directions:

1. In your slow cooker, combine the chickpeas with the stock, salt, pepper, and garlic, stir, put the lid on and cook on Low for 8 hours.

2. Drain chickpeas, transfer them to a blender, add the rest of the ingredients, pulse well, divide into bowls and serve as a party spread.

Corn Dip

Ingredients:

- 2 tablespoon salt
- 1/2 cup Worcestershire sauce
- 2 teaspoon garlic powder
- 10 cups corn, rice, and wheat cereal
- 2 cup cheerios
- 2 cups pretzels
- 2 cup peanuts
- 6 tablespoons hot, melted butter

Directions:

1. In your slow cooker, mix cereal with cheerios, pretzels, peanuts, butter, salt, Worcestershire sauce, and garlic powder, toss well, cover, and cook on Low for 4 hours.

2. Divide into bowls and serve as a snack.

Spinach Dip

Ingredients:

- 1 pound baby spinach
- 2 garlic cloves, minced
- Salt and black pepper to the taste
- 2 tablespoons heavy cream
- 1 cup Greek yogurt

Directions:

1. In your slow cooker, mix the spinach with the cream and the other ingredients, toss, put the lid on and cook on High for 2 hour.

2. Blend using an immersion blender, divide into bowls and serve as a party dip.

Candied Pecans

Ingredients:

- 1 cup brown sugar
- 2 fresh egg white, whisked
- 4 cups pecans
- 2 teaspoons vanilla extract
- 1/2 cup water
- 2 cup white sugar
- 2 and 1 tablespoons cinnamon powder

Directions:

1. In a bowl, mix white sugar with cinnamon, brown sugar, and vanilla and stir.

2. Dip pecans in fresh egg white, then in the sugar mix and put them in your slow cooker, also add the water, cover and cook on Low for 4 hours.

3. Divide into bowls and serve as a snack.

Dill Potato Salad

Ingredients:

- 1 cup heavy cream
- 2 tablespoons mustard
- A pinch of salt and black pepper
- 2 tablespoon dill, chopped
- 1 cup celery, chopped
- 2 red onion, sliced

- 2 pound gold potatoes, peeled and roughly cubed
- 2 tablespoons balsamic vinegar

Directions:

1. In your slow cooker, mix the potatoes with the cream, mustard, and the other ingredients, toss, put the lid on and cook on Low for 8 hours.

2. Divide salad into bowls and serve as an appetizer.

Chicken Bites

Ingredients:

- 2 pound chicken thighs, boneless and skinless

- 2 and 1 cups chicken stock

- 2 tablespoons lemon juice

- 1 cup green olives, pitted and roughly chopped

- Salt to the taste

- 4 tablespoons olive oil

- 6 pita breads, cut in quarters and heated in the oven

- 2 tablespoon ginger, grated

- 2 yellow onion, sliced

- 2 tablespoon garlic, minced

- 2 teaspoons cumin, ground

- 2 teaspoon cinnamon powder

- 2 tablespoons sweet paprika

Directions:

1. Heat up a pan with the olive oil over medium-high heat, add onions, garlic, ginger, salt, and pepper, stir and cook for 5 minutes.

2. Add cumin and cinnamon, stir well and take off the heat.

3. Put chicken pieces in your slow cooker, add onions mix, lemon juice, olives, and

stock, stir, cover, and cook on Low for 8 hours.

4. Shred meat, stir the whole mixture again, divide it on pita chips, and serve as a snack.

Peanut Snack

Ingredients:

- 1 ounces dark chocolate chips
- 1 ounces white chocolate chips
- 2 cup peanuts
- 2 cup chocolate peanut butter

Directions:

1. In your slow cooker, mix peanuts with peanut butter, dark and white chocolate chips, cover, and cook on Low for 2 hour and 45 minutes.

2. Divide this mix into small muffin cups, leave aside to cool down, and serve as a snack.

Apple Dip

Ingredients:

- 1 ounces jarred caramel sauce

- A pinch of nutmeg, ground

- 6 apples, peeled and chopped

- 1 teaspoon cinnamon powder

Directions:

1. In your slow cooker, mix apples with cinnamon, caramel sauce, and nutmeg, stir, cover and cook on High for 2 hour and 45 minutes.

2. Divide into bowls and serve.

Tomato And Mushroom Salsa

Ingredients:

- 2 garlic clove, minced
- 1 ounces tomato sauce
- 1/2 cup cream cheese, cubed
- 2 tablespoon chives, chopped
- Salt and black pepper to the taste
- 2 cup cherry tomatoes, halved
- 2 cup mushrooms, sliced
- 2 small yellow onion, chopped

Directions:

1. In your slow cooker, mix the tomatoes with the mushrooms and the other ingredients, toss, put the lid on and cook on Low for 4 hours.

2. Divide into bowls and serve as a party salsa

Delicious Apple Crisp

Ingredients:

- 1/2 tsp ground nutmeg
- 1 tsp ground cinnamon
- 1/2 cup brown sugar
- 1/2 cup flour
- 1/2 cup old-fashioned oats
- 2 lbs apples, peeled & sliced
- 1 cup butter

Directions:

1. Add sliced apples into the cooking pot.

2. In a mixing bowl, mix together flour, nutmeg, cinnamon, sugar, and oats.

3. Add butter into the flour mixture and mix until the mixture is crumbly.

4. Sprinkle flour mixture over sliced apples.

5. Cover instant pot aura with lid.

6. Select slow cook mode and cook on High for 2-4 hours.

7. Top with vanilla ice-cream and serve.

Easy Peach Cobbler Cake

Ingredients:

- 25 oz can pineapples, crushed
- 22 oz can peach pie filling
- 1/3 cup butter, cut into pieces
- 2 oz yellow cake mix

Directions:

1. Pour crushed pineapples and peach pie filling into the cooking pot and spread evenly.

2. Sprinkle cake mix on top of pineapple mixture, then places butter pieces on top of the cake mix.

3. Cover instant pot aura with lid.

4. Select Bake mode and set the temperature to 480 F and time for 50 minutes.

5. Serve with vanilla ice cream.

Strawberry Dump Cake

Ingredients:

- 25 oz can pineapple, crushed
- 1 /2 cups strawberries, frozen, thawed, & sliced
- 30 oz box cake mix

Directions:

1. Add strawberries into the cooking pot and spread evenly.
2. Mix together cake mix and crushed pineapple and pour over sliced strawberries and spread evenly.
3. Cover instant pot aura with lid.
4. Select Bake mode and set the temperature to 480 F and time for 45 minutes.

5. Serve and enjoy.

Baked Apples

Ingredients:

- 2 tbsp butter, melted
- 4 apples, sliced
- 1 tsp cinnamon

Directions:

1. Toss sliced apples with butter and cinnamon and place them into the cooking pot.

2. Cover instant pot aura with lid.

3. Select Bake mode and set the temperature to 490 F and time for 45 minutes.

4. Serve and enjoy.

Baked Peaches

Ingredients:

- 2 tbsp brown sugar

- 2 tbsp butter

- 4 ripe peaches, slice in half & remove the pit

- 1/2 tsp cinnamon

Directions:

1. Mix together butter, brown sugar, and cinnamon and place in the middle of each peach piece.

2. Place peaches in the cooking pot.

3. Cover instant pot aura with lid.

4. Select Bake mode and set the temperature to 490 F and time for 25 minutes.

5. Serve and enjoy.

Delicious Peach Crisp

Ingredients:

- 5 cups rolled oats
- 2 tbsp cornstarch
- 1 cup sugar
- 8 cups can peach, sliced
- 1 cup butter, cubed
- 1 cup brown sugar
- 1 cup all-purpose flour

Directions:

1. Add peaches, cornstarch, and sugar into the cooking pot and stir well.

2. Mix together butter, brown sugar, flour, and oats and sprinkle over peaches.

3. Cover instant pot aura with lid.

4. Select Bake mode and set the temperature to 480 F and time for 45 - 50 minutes.

5. Serve with ice cream

Marinated Mushrooms

Ingredients:

- 2 teaspoon of Worcestershire sauce
- 2 teaspoon of garlic powder
- 4 lbs. fresh mushrooms
- 1 cup of butter, or more as needed
- 4 cubes beef bouillon
- 2 cups of boiling water
- 2 cup of dry red wine
- 2 teaspoon of dill weed

Directions:

1. Start by throwing all the Ingredients: into the Crockpot.
2. Cover its lid and cook for 1 hours on Low setting.
3. Once done, remove its lid of the crockpot carefully.
4. Mix well and garnish as desired.
5. Serve warm.

Masala Broccoli

Ingredients:

- 2 spring onions, chopped
- 2 teaspoon curry powder
- 1 teaspoon chili pepper
- 1 cup organic almond milk
- 2 cups broccoli florets
- 2 tablespoon garam masala

Directions:

1. In the slow cooker, mix the broccoli with the masala and the other ingredients.
2. Close the lid and cook korma for 6 hours on low.
3. Divide between plates and serve.

Chard And Radishes

Ingredients:

- 2 teaspoon salt
- 1/2 teaspoon ground ginger
- 1/2 cup veggie stock
- 2 cups red chard, torn
- 2 cup radishes, halved
- 2 teaspoon sweet paprika
- 1/2 cup butter

Directions:

1. In the slow cooker, mix the chard with radishes and the other ingredients
2. Close the slow cooker lid and cook the beet greens for 4 hours on High.
3. Mix up the mix carefully before serving.

Bbq Smokies

Ingredients:

- 1/2 cup of diced onion
- 2 packages little wieners
- 2 cup of sugar-free tomato sauce
- 2 tablespoon of Worcestershire sauce

Directions:

1. Start by throwing all the Ingredients: into the Crockpot.
2. Cover its lid and cook for 2 hours on Low setting.
3. Once done, remove its lid of the crockpot carefully.
4. Mix well and garnish as desired.
5. Serve warm.

Cranberry Brussels Sprouts Mix

Ingredients:

- 2 teaspoons of thyme, diced
- 2 cup of cranberries, dried
- 4 tablespoon of olive oil
- 2 teaspoons of rosemary, diced
- 2 tablespoons of balsamic vinegar

Directions:

1. Start by throwing all the Ingredients: into the Crockpot.
2. Cover its lid and cook for 4 hours on Low setting.
3. Once done, remove its lid of the crockpot carefully.
4. Mix well and garnish as desired.
5. Serve warm.

Zucchini Slices With Mozzarella

Ingredients:

- 2 teaspoon butter
- 2 tablespoon coconut flakes, unsweetened
- 2 teaspoon minced garlic
- 4 oz Mozzarella, sliced
- 2 zucchini, sliced
- 2 tablespoon olive oil

Directions:

1. Sprinkle the zucchini slices with the olive oil, coconut flakes, and minced garlic.

2. Place the zucchini slices in a flat layer on the bottom of the slow cooker along with the butter.
3. Place a piece of mozzarella on top of each zucchini slice.
4. Close the lid and cook the meal for 2 hour on High.
5. Serve hot!

Kale Mash With Blue Cheese

Ingredients:

- 2 tablespoon butter
- 2 teaspoon salt
- 2 teaspoon ground black pepper
- 4 oz Blue cheese
- 2 cup Italian dark-leaf kale
- ¾ cup almond milk, unsweetened

Directions:

1. Chop the kale and place it in the slow cooker.
2. Add almond milk, salt, and ground black pepper.
3. Close the lid and cook the kale for 6 hours on Low.
4. Meanwhile, chop Blue cheese and butter.
5. Combine the cooked kale with the butter and stir it until butter is melted.

6. Add the Blue cheese and stir it gently.
7. Serve!

Cheesy Spaghetti Squash

Ingredients:

- 1 teaspoon thyme
- 2 teaspoon paprika
- 1/2 cup water
- 2 oz Parmesan, sliced
- 25 oz spaghetti squash, peeled and seeded
- 2 tablespoon butter

Directions:

1. Grate the spaghetti squash and place it in the slow cooker.
2. Add the butter, thyme, paprika, and water.
3. Stir the mixture gently with a spoon.

4. Then cover the squash with the sliced cheese and close the lid.
5. Cook the meal for 4 hours on Low.
6. Let the cooked squash rest for 35 minutes.
7. Serve it!

Thai Cabbage

Ingredients:

- 4 tablespoons water
- 2 teaspoon salt
- 4 tablespoons butter, melted
- 2 tablespoon coconut oil
- 8 oz white cabbage, shredded
- 2 tablespoon curry paste

Directions:

1. Mix the curry paste and water.
2. Add salt and coconut oil and whisk.

3. Place the shredded cabbage in the slow cooker.
4. Sprinkle it with the curry paste mixture.
5. Add the butter and stir the vegetables gently.
6. Close the lid and cook the cabbage on Low for 6 hours.
7. When the time is done, let the cabbage rest for 25 minutes.
8. Serve it!

Flax Meal Coffeecake

Ingredients:

- 1 cup flax seed meal
- 1 teaspoon baking soda
- ¾ cup powdered Swerve, divided 2 teaspoons vanilla extract, divided
- 2 teaspoons cinnamon
- 1 cup of warm water
- 2 Tablespoon butter for the crock-pot
- 25 eggs
- ¾ cup coconut flour
- 2 tablespoon gelatin
- 2 cup butter, divided

Directions:

1. Butter the crock-pot.
2. In a blender, mix the eggs, flour, 1 cup butter, sweetener, gelatin and vanilla. Blend for 25 seconds.

3. In a small bowl, mix flax meal and baking soda.
4. Add to mixture in blender.
5. Blend for 25 seconds.
6. Combine 1 cup melted butter, sweetener, water, and cinnamon to make a syrup; add a bit of water, if not liquid enough.
7. Pour 2 layer of batter in the buttered crock-pot.
8. Sprinkle with 1/2 of the syrup.
9. Repeat two more times, finishing with 1 of the syrup.
10.   Cover the crock-pot with a paper towel to absorb the water.
11.   Cover, cook on low for 4 hours.

Lime Zucchini Noodles

Ingredients:

- 1/2 teaspoon sweet paprika
- 1 teaspoon salt
- 1/2 cup water
- 2 teaspoon butter
- 8 oz zucchini noodles
- 2 tablespoon balsamic vinegar
- 2 tablespoon lime juice

Directions:

1. In the slow cooker, mix the noodles with the vinegar and the other ingredients.
2. Put the lid on and cook noodles for4 hours on Low.
3. Divide between plates and serve.

Pumpkin Cubes

Ingredients:

- 2 teaspoon butter
- 2 tablespoons water
- 2 teaspoon ground ginger
- 8 oz pumpkin
- 2 teaspoon ground cinnamon
- 2 teaspoon liquid stevia

Directions:

1. Peel the pumpkin and chop it.
2. Place the chopped pumpkin in the slow cooker.
3. Add ground cinnamon, liquid stevia, and ground ginger.
4. Stir it gently and add water and butter.
5. Close the lid and cook the pumpkin for 6 hours on Low.
6. When the pumpkin is cooked, it will be nice and tender.

7. Let it rest for 25 minutes.
8. Enjoy!

Cowboy Mexican Dip

Ingredients:

- 2   can tomatoes and green chilis
- 2 loaf processed cheese, cubed
- 2 can chili

Directions:

1. Start by throwing all the Ingredients: into the Crockpot.
2. Cover its lid and cook for 2 hours on Low setting.
3. Once done, remove its lid of the crockpot carefully.
4. Mix well and garnish as desired.
5. Serve warm.

Celery Puree

Ingredients:

- 2 teaspoon sweet paprika
- 2 teaspoon chives, chopped
- 1 cup of water
- 2 cup celery stalks, chopped
- 2 tablespoons butter

Directions:

1. Put celery and water in the slow cooker.
2. Close the lid and cook it for 4 hours on High.
3. Then drain water and mash until you get soft mash.
4. Add the rest of the ingredients, whisk and serve.

Garlicky Mashed Cauliflower

Ingredients:

- 4 Tablespoons of butter
- ⅓ cup sour cream
- 4 Tablespoons combined fresh chopped herbs: chives, parsley or spring onions
- Salt and pepper
- 2 good-sized head of cauliflower, cut into florets
- 2 small head of garlic, peeled
- 4 cups vegetable broth

Directions:

1. Place the cauliflower, garlic in the crock-pot.
2. Pour in broth until cauliflower is covered.
3. Add more liquid, if needed.
4. Cover, cook on high for 4 hours.

5. Drain the liquid, reserving for later.
6. Mash the vegetables with a fork or a potato masher.
7. Add the cream and butter and mash again until smooth.
8. If necessary, add some of the reserved cooking liquid to soften the mash.
9. Mix in chopped herbs, add salt and fresh ground pepper.
10.   Stir to combine thoroughly.

Tomato And Spaghetti Squash

Ingredients:

- 2 teaspoon butter
- 1 teaspoon garlic powder
- 1 teaspoon turmeric powder
- 1 cup of water
- 25 oz spaghetti squash, halved
- 2 cup cherry tomatoes, halved
- 2 teaspoon sweet paprika
- 2 oz Parmesan

Directions:

1. Pour water in the slow cooker.
2. Add spaghetti squash and cook it on High for 4 hours.
3. When the squash is soft, it is cooked.
4. Shred the vegetable with the help of the fork.

5. In the shallow bowl, mix the spaghetti squash with the remaining ingredients, toss and serve.

Rhubarb And Zucchini Mix

Ingredients:

- 2 teaspoon garam masala
- 8 oz Cheddar cheese, shredded
- 4 tablespoons coconut cream
- 2 teaspoon butter
- 2 teaspoon olive oil
- 1 teaspoon salt
- 1/2 cup fresh cilantro, chopped
- 2 cups rhubarb, chopped
- 2 cup zucchini, sliced
- 2 teaspoon coriander, ground
- 2 teaspoon curry powder

Directions:

1. In the slow cooker, mix the rhubarb with the zucchini and the other ingredients, toss and close the slow cooker lid.
2. Cook the mix for 6 hours on Low.

Coconut Kale

Ingredients:

- 2 teaspoon almonds, crushed
- 2 teaspoon butter
- 1 teaspoon turmeric
- 25 oz Italian dark-leaf kale
- 2   tablespoon   coconut   flakes, unsweetened
- 1 cup coconut milk, unsweetened

Directions:

1. Chop the kale and place it in the slow cooker.
2. Add the coconut milk, butter, and turmeric.
3. Close the lid and cook the kale for 45 minutes on High.
4. Transfer the kale to serving plates.
5. Sprinkle with the crushed almonds and coconut flakes.

6. Serve it!

Artichoke And Broccoli Mix

Ingredients:

- 4 tablespoons olive oil
- 1 teaspoon salt
- 1 garlic clove, minced
- 1/2 cup water
- 4 tablespoons lemon juice
- 2 artichokes, trimmed and halved
- 2 cup broccoli florets
- 2 teaspoon tahini paste
- 1 teaspoon sweet paprika

Directions:

1. In the slow cooker, mix the artichokes with the broccoli and the other ingredients and close the lid.
2. Cook the vegetable for 6 hours on Low.

3. Divide between plates and serve.

Zucchini And Radish Mix

Ingredients:

- 2 tablespoon butter
- 1 teaspoon salt
- 1 teaspoon ground black pepper
- 2 tablespoon chives, chopped
- 2 zucchinis, trimmed and sliced
- 2 cup radishes, halved
- 1/2 cup of veggie stock

Directions:

1. In the slow cooker, combine all the ingredients and toss gently.
2. Close the slow cooker lid and cook a meal for 2 hours on Low.

Eggplant Hash

Ingredients:

- 1 cup water
- 2 oz butter
- 2 teaspoon cayenne pepper
- 2 eggplants, peeled, chopped
- 2 onion, diced
- 6 oz white mushrooms, chopped

Directions:

1. Place the eggplants and onion in the slow cooker.
2. Sprinkle the vegetables with the chopped mushrooms, water, butter, and cayenne pepper.
3. Stir the vegetable gently and close the lid.
4. Cook the eggplants hash for 4 hours on High.

5. When the eggplants hash is cooked, let it chill for 25 minutes.
6. Serve it!

Spiced Fennel Slices

Ingredients:

- 2 teaspoon salt
- 2 oz butter
- 2 tablespoon olive oil
- 2 -pound fennel bulb
- 2 teaspoon cumin
- 2 teaspoon thyme

Directions:

1. Mix the cumin, thyme, salt, and olive oil.
2. Slice the fennel bulb and sprinkle it with the spice mixture.
3. Place the fennel in the slow cooker and add butter.
4. Close the lid and cook for 2 hours on High.
5. Serve the meal hot!

Cauliflower Croquettes

Ingredients:

- 4 tablespoons almond flour
- 2 tablespoon butter
- 1 teaspoon cayenne pepper
- 2 fresh egg
- 8 oz cauliflower, grated
- 2 teaspoon salt

Directions:

1. Beat the fresh egg in a bowl.
2. Add grated cauliflower, salt, and cayenne pepper to the whisked fresh egg and stir.
3. Then make small balls from the mixture and coat them with the almond flour.
4. Toss the butter in the slow cooker.
5. Add the cauliflower croquettes to the slow cooker as well and cook them for 2 hours on High.

6. Let the cooked croquettes cool for at least 25 minutes.
7. Serve!

Sautéed Bell Peppers

Ingredients:

- ¾ cup coconut milk, unsweetened
- 2 teaspoon butter
- 2 teaspoon thyme
- 2 onion, diced
- 2 teaspoon turmeric
- 8 oz bell peppers
- 8 oz cauliflower, chopped
- 2 oz bacon, chopped
- 2 teaspoon salt
- 2 teaspoon ground black pepper

Directions:

1. Remove the seeds from the bell peppers and chop them roughly.
2. Place the bell peppers, cauliflower, and bacon in the slow cooker.
3. Add the salt, ground black pepper, coconut milk, butter, milk, and thyme.

4. Stir well then add the diced onion.
5. Add the turmeric and stir the mixture.
6. Close the lid and cook 6 hours on Low.
7. When the meal is cooked, let it chill for 25 minutes and serve it!

Mint Peppers

Ingredients:

- 2 teaspoons mint, dried
- 2 teaspoon curry powder
- 1 teaspoon turmeric
- 2 teaspoon chili flakes
- 1/2 cup of water
- 1 cup crushed tomatoes
- 2 green bell peppers, roughly chopped
- 2 red bell peppers, roughly chopped

Directions:

1. In the slow cooker, mix the peppers with tomatoes and the other ingredients.
2. Close the slow cooker lid and cook for 8 hours on Low.
3. Divide into bowls and serve.

Brussel Sprouts With Parmesan

Ingredients:

- ¾ cup water
- 1/2 teaspoon minced garlic
- 2 teaspoon dried oregano
- 10 oz Brussel sprouts
- 4 oz Parmesan, sliced

Directions:

1. Place Brussel sprouts in the slow cooker.
2. Add the minced garlic and dried oregano.
3. Add the water and cook the vegetables for 4 hours on Low.
4. Strain the Brussel sprouts and place them back in the slow cooker.
5. Add the sliced cheese and cook it for 45 minutes more on High.
6. Enjoy!

Paprika Spaghetti Squash

Ingredients:

- 2 tablespoon rosemary, chopped
- 1 teaspoon curry powder
- 2 teaspoon onion powder
- 2 teaspoon garlic powder
- 1/2 cup chicken stock
- 2 -pound spaghetti squash, shredded
- 2 teaspoon ground paprika
- 2 teaspoon smoked paprika
- 2 teaspoon salt

Directions:

1. In the slow cooker, mix the squash with paprika and the other ingredients, toss and close the lid.
2. Cook it for 4.6 hours on Low.
3. Divide between plates and serve.

Eggplant Gratin

Ingredients:

- 2 tablespoon dried parsley
- 4 oz Parmesan, grated
- 4 tablespoons water
- 2 teaspoon chili flakes
- 2 tablespoon butter
- 2 teaspoon minced garlic
- 2 eggplants, chopped
- 2 teaspoon salt

Directions:

1. Mix the dried parsley, chili flakes, and salt together.
2. Sprinkle the chopped eggplants with the spice mixture and stir well.
3. Place the eggplants in the slow cooker.
4. Add the water and minced garlic.
5. Add the butter and sprinkle with the grated Parmesan.

6. Close the lid and cook the gratin for 6 hours on Low.
7. Open the lid and cool the gratin for 25 minutes.
8. Serve it.

Okra And Artichokes

Ingredients:

- 2 tablespoons chives, chopped
- 2 teaspoon ground black pepper
- ¾ cup heavy cream
- 10 oz okra, sliced
- 2 artichokes, trimmed and quartered
- 2 jalapeno, sliced

Directions:

1. In the slow cooker, mix the okra with the artichokes and the other ingredients,
2. Close the slow cooker lid and cook the mix for 6 hours on Low.

Okra Stew

Ingredients:

- 2 teaspoon butter
- 2 teaspoon paprika
- 1 teaspoon ground black pepper
- 2 teaspoon dried dill
- 25 oz okra, chopped
- 2 onion, diced
- 6 oz cauliflower, chopped
- 2 cup water

Directions:

1. Mix the chopped okra, diced onion, cauliflower, and spices.
2. Stir the mixture and place it in the slow cooker.
3. Add water and butter and close the lid.
4. Cook the stew for 6 hours on Low.
5. Transfer the dish into serving bowls and serve!

Layered Mushrooms

Ingredients:

- 2 teaspoon cayenne pepper
- 2 onion, grated
- 6 tablespoons almond milk, unsweetened
- 2 oz butter
- 8 oz white mushrooms, sliced
- 2 eggplant, peeled, sliced
- 2 tablespoon dried dill

Directions:

1. Mix the dried dill, cayenne pepper, and butter.
2. Stir the mixture until smooth.
3. Melt the butter mixture.
4. Make a layer of the slice eggplant in the slow cooker.
5. Brush it with some of the butter mixture.

6. Make the layer of the mushrooms and top it with the grated onion.
7. Add all the remaining butter mixture and almond milk.
8. Close the lid and cook the meal for 6 hours on Low.
9. Let the cooked mushrooms rest for 30 - 25 minutes.
   10.   Serve!

Eggplants And Olives

Ingredients:

- 1 cup keto marinara sauce
- 2 tablespoon cilantro, chopped
- 2 teaspoon salt
- 2 teaspoon dried oregano
- 4 eggplants, trimmed and roughly cubed
- 1 cup black olives, pitted and halved

Directions:

1. In the slow cooker, mix the eggplants with the olives and the other ingredients.
2. Close the lid and cook the dish for 4 hours on High.

Glazed Spiced Carrots

Ingredients:

- 1/2 teaspoon of salt
- 2 /8 teaspoon of ground nutmeg
- 2 tablespoons of xanthan gum
- 2 tablespoons of water
- Toasted diced pecans,
- 1 cup of peach preserves
- 1 cup of butter, melted
- 1/2 cup of packed brown swerve
- 2 teaspoon of vanilla extract
- 1 teaspoon of cinnamon, ground

Directions:

1. Start by throwing all the Ingredients: into the Crockpot.
2. Cover its lid and cook for 8 hours on Low setting.
3. Once done, remove its lid of the crockpot carefully.

4. Mix well and garnish as desired.
5. Serve warm.

Oregano Green Beans

Ingredients:

- 2 teaspoon rosemary, dried
- 2 teaspoon salt
- ¾ teaspoon dried oregano
- 2 cups green beans, trimmed and halved
- 1 cup coconut cream
- 2 teaspoon turmeric powder

Directions:

1. In the slow cooker, mix the peas with the cream and the other ingredients.
2. Close the slow cooker lid and cook for 6 hours on Low.
3. Divide between plates and serve.

Curry Cauliflower

Ingredients:

- 1 teaspoon dried cilantro
- 2 oz butter
- ¾ cup water
- 1/2 cup chicken stock
- 25 oz cauliflower
- 2 teaspoon curry paste
- 2 teaspoon curry powder

Directions:

1. Chop the cauliflower roughly and sprinkle it with the curry powder and dried cilantro.
2. Place the chopped cauliflower in the slow cooker.
3. Mix the curry paste with the water.
4. Add chicken stock and transfer the liquid to the slow cooker.
5. Add butter and close the lid.

6. Cook the cauliflower for 6 hours on Low.
7. Strain 1 of the liquid off and discard. Transfer the cauliflower to serving bowls.
8. Serve it!

Halibut Fillets In Romaine Leaves

Ingredients:

- 2 halibut steaks, 4 ounces each
- 1 tsp dried tarragon leaves
- 1 cup dry white wine or chicken broth
- 6 large romaine leaves
  - Salt
  - Pepper
- 1/2 cup thinly sliced spinach

Instructions:

1. Put the wine or chicken broth in the slow cooker.

2. Cover and cook for 35 minutes on high.

3. Slice off the large centre vein from the romaine leaves, but make sure that the leaves are still intact.

4. Plunge them in boiling water for approximately 45 seconds, or until wilted.

5. Drain thoroughly.

6. Season the halibut steaks with the tarragon leaves, salt and pepper.

7. Sprinkle the spinach on top then wrap the fish in romaine leaves, with three leaves per fish.

8. Arrange the fish, seam sides down, in the slow cooker.

9. Cover and cook for 2 hour on high or until the fish is well done.

10. Serve immediately.

Seafood Veracruz

Ingredients:

- 4 Tbsp tomato paste

- 1 cup sliced green olives

- 4 lb red snapper or other firm white fish fillets, sliced into 8 pieces

- Sea salt

- Freshly ground black pepper

- 4 onions, sliced thinly

- 4 Tbsp olive oil

- 2 Serrano chilies or jalapeno, seeded and minced

- 4 tsp dried oregano

- 2 Tbsp chili powder

- 45 oz dice tomatoes, undrained

- 2 cups seafood stock

- 2 tsp grated lemon zest
- 4 Tbsp freshly squeezed lemon juice

Instructions:

1. Place a skillet over fresh high flame and heat the oil.

2. Sauté the onion, chili, and garlic until onion is translucent.

3. Reduce to low flame, then add the oregano and chili powder.

4. Sauté for 2 minute, then transfer to the slow cooker.

5. Add the lemon juice and zest, stock, tomatoes, and tomato paste into the slow cooker.

6. Combine thoroughly.

7. Cover and cook for 6 hours on low or for 4 hours on high.

8. Set heat to high, then add the olives and fish.

9. Cover and cook for 45 minutes, or until fish is cooked through.

10. Season with salt and pepper to taste, then serve.

Salmon Loaf With Cucumber Sauce

Ingredients:

- 2 /8 cup chopped green onion

- 2 /8 cup almond milk

- 4 ounces canned salmon, drained

- 1 cup fresh gluten free "bread" crumbs

  2 fresh egg

- 2 /8 tsp pepper

- 1/2 cup coconut cream

- 1/2 cup chopped cucumber

- 1/2 tsp dill weed

- 2 Tbsp lemon juice

- 2 Tbsp capers

- 1 Tbsp dried dill weed

- 1/2 tsp salt

- Salt
- White pepper

Instructions:

1. Line the insert of the slow cooker with aluminum foil.

2. Make sure that the ends are sticking out so that you can use them to pull up the foil "basket" later on.

3. In a bowl, mix together the salmon, gluten-free crumbs, green onion, almond milk, egg, lemon juice, capers, dill, salt, and pepper.

4. Pack the mixture in the lined slow cooker.

5. Cover and cook for 4 hours on low, then take out the loaf by pulling the foil basket out.

6. Make the cucumber sauce by mixing the coconut cream, cucumber, and dill.

7. Season with salt and pepper.

8. Slice the salmon loaf and serve with the cucumber sauce.

Caribbean Fish Curry

Ingredients:

- 2 Tbsp ground cumin

- 45 oz canned light coconut milk

- 4 cups frozen or fresh peas, thawed

- 4 1 lb grouper or other thick white fish, rinsed and cubed

- Sea salt

- Freshly ground black pepper

- 4 Tbsp olive oil

- 8 garlic cloves, minced

- 4 fresh onions, diced

- 2 jalapeno or Scotch bonnet chilies, seeded and minced

- 6 ripe plum tomatoes, seeded and diced

- 4 Tbsp curry powder

Instructions:

1. Heat the oil over fresh high flame in a skillet.

2. Sauté the onion, chilies, and garlic until onion is translucent.

3. Reduce to low flame, then add the cumin and curry powder.

4. Sauté for 2 minute, then transfer to the slow cooker.

5. Add the coconut milk and tomatoes into the slow cooker.

6. Cover and cook for 8 hours on low or for 4 hours on high.

7. Set heat to high, then add the peas and fish.

8. Cover and cook for 45 minutes, or until fish is cooked through.

9. Season with salt and pepper to taste, then serve at once.

Poached Haddock

Ingredients:

- 2 cup fish stock
- 30 oz unsalted tomato sauce
- 2 tsp minced garlic
- 1/2 tsp cumin
- 4 Tbsp lemon juice
- 4 lb haddock
- 2 Tbsp olive oil
- 2 cups finely chopped onion

Instructions:

1. Place a skillet over fresh flame and heat the olive oil.

2. Sauté the onion until translucent, then add the fish stock and bring to a boil.

3. Pour the onion and fish stock mixture into the slow cooker.

4. Add the tomato sauce, garlic, lemon juice and cumin.

5. Stir to combine then cover and cook for 2 hours on high to a simmer.

6. Add the haddock into the slow cooker and cook for 2 hour or until tender and cooked through. Serve hot.

Shrimp Creole

Ingredients:

- 2 1/3 cups chopped onion
- 1 oz unsalted tomato sauce
- 4 2 oz unsalted whole tomatoes, torn
- 1/3 tsp minced garlic
- 1 drops hot pepper sauce
- 1 tsp black pepper
- 5 lb shrimp, peeled and deveined
- 2 cups sliced celery
- 5 cups chopped green bell pepper

Instructions:

1. Stir together the celery, bell pepper, onion, tomatoes, tomato sauce, garlic, hot sauce and black pepper in the slow cooker.

2. Cover and cook for 2 hours on high or for 6 hours on low.

3. Stir in the shrimp, cover and cook for an additional 2 hour.

4. Serve immediately.

Savory Orange Chicken

Ingredients:

- 2 clove garlic, minced
- 2 /8 cup water
- 2 small onion, quartered
- 5 Tbsp orange juice
- 1/2 cup non fat Greek yogurt
- 1/2 cup almonds, chopped
- 2 lbs chopped chicken breast
- 1/2 cup chicken broth
- 1 lb asparagus, sliced into bite sized pieces
- 1 bell pepper, chopped
- 1 tsp dried thyme

Instructions:

1. Combine the garlic, onion, and pepper in the slow cooker and add the orange juice and chicken broth.

2. Stir in the thyme and arrange the chicken inside, turning the pieces to coat.

3. Cover the slow cooker and cook for 4 hours on low.

4. Stir in the asparagus and the water.

5. Cover and cook for an additional hour or until the asparagus is fork tender.

6. Spoon the dish onto plates.

7. Add a dollop of yogurt over each dish and sprinkle the almonds on top.

8. Serve immediately.

Kale And Chicken Stew

Ingredients:

- 6 cups chopped fresh kale
- 1 cup cream cheese
- 5 tsp salt
- 5 tsp garlic powder
- 1/3 tsp black pepper
- Water, as needed
- 6 chicken breasts, sliced into chunks
- 4 cups diced tomatoes with juices
- 2 cup black beans, soaked overnight
- 2 large onion, sliced thinly into strips

Instructions:

1. Combine the beans, chicken, tomatoes with juices, onion, kale, garlic powder, salt and pepper in the slow cooker.

2. Add just enough water to cover the ingredients.

3. Cover and cook for 4 hours on low, stirring once every hour or so.

4. Stir in the cream cheese and cook for an additional half hour on low.

5. Ladle into soup bowls and serve immediately

Lemon Ginger Turkey

Ingredients:

- 2 small onions, chopped
- 4 tsp coconut oil
- 2 cups diced tomatoes with juices
- 1 cup lemon juice
- 5 lb turkey breast
- 4 cloves garlic, minced
- 5 cups chicken broth
- 4 inches fresh ginger, peeled and grated
- Salt
- 2 lemon, sliced into 6 wedges
- Black pepper

Instructions:

1. Season the turkey all over with salt and black pepper.

2. Place a saucepan over fresh flame and heat 2 teaspoon of coconut oil.

3. Brown the turkey all over, then set aside on a plate.

4. Place the saucepan back over fresh flame and heat 1 teaspoon of coconut oil.

5. Sauté the onion until browned then set aside.

6. Place the remaining coconut oil in the slow cooker and add the garlic, ginger, browned onion, turkey, chicken broth and lemon juice.

7. Stir well to combine and season to taste with salt and pepper.

8. Cover the slow cooker and cook on fresh heat for 2 hour.

9. Stir in the tomatoes with the juices.

10.   Cover and cook for 4 hours on low.

11.   Divide the turkey dish among 6 plates and serve with a lemon wedge.

Creamy Buttered Chicken

Ingredients:

- 1/3 cup butter

- 2 large onion, diced

- 5 cups non-fat Greek yogurt

- 4 cloves garlic, minced

- 4 Tbsp coconut oil

- 6 chicken thighs

- 5 cups diced tomatoes

- 5 cups tomato sauce

- 2 cup coconut milk

- Salt

- Black pepper

Instructions:

1. Place a skillet over fresh flame and melt the butter and coconut oil together.

2. Stir to combine.

3. Sauté the onion and garlic until onion becomes translucent.

4. Add the chicken and cook until browned, then stir in the tomato paste and cook until heated through.

5. Pour the chicken mixture into the slow cooker and add the diced tomatoes, yogurt and coconut milk.

6. Season to taste with salt and pepper.

7. Cover and cook on low for 8 hours, adding more water if needed to keep the sauce from drying out.

8. Transfer the chicken thighs onto a platter and ladle the sauce on top.

9. Serve immediately.

Brandied Vanilla Bean Applesauce

Ingredients:

- 2 Tbsp raw honey or maple syrup

- 2 Tbsp brandy

- 1/2 vanilla bean, sliced lengthwise

- 2 cup organic apple juice

- 6   sweet tart apples ● 5 Tbsp coconut oil or ghee, melted

Instructions:

1. Pour the apple juice into a mixing bowl.

2. Peel the apples and remove the core.

3. Thinly slice them and place them into the apple juice instantly to prevent them from becoming brown.

4. Drain the apple slices, but make sure to reserve about 5 tablespoons of the apple juice.

5. Put the apple slices back into the emptied mixing bowl and add the 5 tablespoons of apple juice.

6. Add the coconut oil or ghee, raw honey or maple syrup, and brandy.

7. Toss to coat.

8. Scrape the mixture into a 2 quart slow cooker and push the vanilla bean deep into the center of the mixture.

9. Cook for 2 hours on low or until the apples are very tender. Take out the vanilla bean and throw it away.

10.   Serve warm or refrigerate in a covered container or serve chilled.

11. You can store it for up to 60 days in the freezer.

Pineapple Coconut Bread Pudding

Ingredients:

- 30 oz canned crushed pineapple, undrained
- 1/2 cup coconut oil, melted
- 1/2 cup rum
- 1/3 tsp pure vanilla extract
- 1/3 lb seed or nut loaf, gluten-free
- Sea salt
- 10 large eggs
- 1/3 cup coconut sugar
- 1 /2 cups coconut milk

- 45 oz canned cream of coconut

Instructions:

1. Cube the loaf into 1 inch pieces. Set aside.

2. Beat the eggs and whisk in the milk, sugar, cream of coconut, coconut oil, rum, and vanilla extract.

3. Add a dash of salt and mix well.

4. Place the cubed loafs into the mixture and press down.

5. Set aside for 25 minutes.

6. Coat the inside of the slow cooker using a nonstick cooking spray.

7. Place the mixture into the slow cooker.

8. Cover and cook for 2 hour on high, then set heat to low and cook for an additional 2 hours and 45 minutes.

9. Internal temperature should be 300degrees F.

10. Serve warm.

Strawberry And Blueberry Crumble

Ingredients:

- 1/2 tsp salt, divided

- 1/2 cup almond or coconut flour, divided

- 2 cups sliced strawberries

- 2 dry pint blueberries

- 1 tsp grated lemon peel

- 1 tsp fresh lemon juice

- 1/2 cup non-contaminated, pure oats

- 4 Tbsp coconut oil or ghee, softened at room temperature

- 1/2 cup light molasses, divided

- 2 /8 tsp ground cinnamon

Instructions:

1. Combine the coconut oil or ghee, half of the molasses, cinnamon, and half of the salt in a mixing bowl.

2. Beat well until smooth.

3. Gradually beat in the oats and half of the flour until thoroughly combined.

4. Cover the bowl with plastic wrap and refrigerate.

5. Meanwhile, wash the strawberries and blueberries.

6. Pat them dry with paper towels and combine them in a large mixing bowl.

7. Add the remaining flour and salt to the berry mixture and toss carefully to coat.

8. Add the lemon juice and grated lemon peel and toss again to coat.

9. Put the mixture into the insert of a 2 quart slow cooker.

10. Take out the cinnamon mixture from the refrigerator and, with clean hands, crumble the cinnamon mixture and sprinkle them on top of the berry mixture in the slow cooker.

11. Cover the slow cooker insert with plastic wrap and refrigerate for approximately 2 hours.

12. Take out the insert from the refrigerator and let it sit at room temperature for half an hour.

13. Take off the plastic wrap and put the insert into the slow cooker.

14. Cover and cook for 2 hour and 45 minutes on low.

15. Once the dessert starts to bubble, serve immediately.

16. You can also set the slow cooker to "warm" for up to an hour before you serve.

Pumpkin Bread

Ingredients:

- 1/3 cup high quality maple syrup
- 5 cup pureed pumpkin
- 2 Tbsp unsweetened almond milk
- 1/3 Tbsp pure vanilla extract
- 1/2 cup chopped toasted pecans
- 5 cups blanched almond flour
- 5 tsp ground cinnamon
- 1/7 tsp ground cinnamon
- 1/3 tsp sea salt
- 1/3 tsp baking soda
- 1/2 cup coconut oil, softened

- 2 fresh eggs

Instructions:

1. Coat the inside of the slow cooker using nonstick cooking spray.

2. Mix together the baking soda, salt, almond flour, nutmeg, and cinnamon in a bowl. Set aside.

3. In another bowl, beat the maple syrup with the coconut oil using an electric mixer, then mix in one fresh egg at a time using low speed.

4. Next, mix in the pumpkin, almond milk, and vanilla extract.

5. Gradually beat the almond flour mixture into the fresh egg mixture until batter is smooth.

6. Pour into the slow cooker, then add the toasted pecans on top, if desired.

7. Cover and cook for 2 hours on high.

8. Insert a toothpick in the center; if it comes out clean, it is ready.

9. Set the bread on a wire rack to cool for at least 25 minutes before slicing.

10. Wrap excess in plastic wrap and place on a cool, dry shelf for up to 8 2 hours.

Dark Chocolate Chip Squares

Ingredients:

- 2 Tbsp maple sugar
- 1/2 tsp baking soda
- 2 cup gluten free baking mix
- Salt
- 2 tsp olive oil
- 1 tsp extract
- 1 cup gluten free, vegan dark chocolate chips
- 1 cup chopped almonds
- 1 cup unsweetened almond or coconut milk
- 2 tsp ground flax seeds
- 4 tsp warm water

Instructions:

1. Line the slow cooker with parchment paper.

2. In a mixing bowl, mix together the baking mix, sugar, baking soda, and salt.

3. In another bowl, mix together the milk, olive oil, and extract.

4. Combine the flax seeds and warm water and stir this into the wet mixture.

5. Combine the dry and wet ingredients together very well, then stir in the chocolate chips and chopped almonds

6. Transfer the mixture into the slow cooker, spreading everything evenly.

7. Place a clean dish towel between the lid and the pot and cook for 50 minutes on high.

8. Remove from the slow cooker and set aside to cool for 25 minutes.

9. Slice into small squares and serve.

Celery And Broccoli Medley

Ingredients:

- 1 cups of vegetable broth
- A pinch of salt and black pepper
- 2 tablespoon of lime juice
- 2 tablespoon of olive oil
- 2 and 1 cups of broccoli florets
- 2 celery stalk, diced

Directions:

1. Start by throwing all the Ingredients: into the Crockpot.
2. Cover its lid and cook for 4 hours on Low setting.
3. Once done, remove its lid of the crockpot carefully.
4. Mix well and garnish as desired.
5. Serve warm.

Salmon

Ingredients:

- Butter, unsalted 2 tablespoon
- Salt 1/2 teaspoon
- Ground black pepper
- 1/2 teaspoon
- Water 1/3 cup
- Salmon fillets 4
- Bunch of dill weed, fresh 2

Directions:

1. Switch on the instant pot, pour in water, stir in lemon juice, and insert a steel steamer rack.
2. Place salmon on the steamer rack, sprinkle with dill and then top with lemon slices.
3. Press the 'keep warm' button, shut the instant pot with its lid in the sealed position, then press the 'manual' button,

press '+/-' to set the cooking time to 6 minutes and cook at high-pressure setting; when the pressure builds in the pot, the cooking timer will start.

4. When the instant pot buzzes, press the 'keep warm' button, do a quick pressure release and open the lid.

5. Remove and discard the lemon slices, transfer salmon to a dish, season with salt and black pepper, garnish with more dill and serve with lemon wedges and cauliflower rice.

Sausage Stew

Ingredients:

- 8 oz sausages, sliced
- 4 spring onions, chopped
- 2 tomato, chopped
- 2 tablespoon Cajun seasonings
- 2 cup of water
- 2 cup keto tomato sauce
- 2 teaspoon minced garlic
- 2 teaspoon olive oil

Directions:

1. In the slow cooker, combine the sausages with the spring onions and the other ingredients and toss.
2. Close the lid and cook gumbo for 4 hours and 45 minutes.

Red Pepper Dip With Warming Spices And Avocado Oil

Ingredients:

- 2 tsp paprika
- 1 tsp cumin
- 1 tsp dried coriander
- 2 lemon
- ¾ cup sour cream
- 6 red peppers seeds and core removed, cut into small chunks
- 4 garlic cloves, crushed
- 2 tsp dried chili flakes

Directions:

1. Drizzle some avocado oil into the Crock Pot.
2. Add the peppers, garlic, all of the spices, salt, pepper, and the finely grated zest of

122

half a lemon to the pot, then add 2 tablespoons of water, stir to combine.

3. Add the lid to the pot and set the temperature to HIGH.

4. Cook for 4 hours or until the capsicum is very soft.

5. Leave to cool slightly.

6. With a hand-held stick blender, blend the peppers until a smooth dip forms.

7. Stir the sour cream and juice of half a lemon into the pepper dip.

8. Serve with a sprinkle of finely chopped fresh parsley and a drizzle of avocado oil.

Cabbage & Corned Beef

Ingredients:

- Allspice
- 2 large head of cabbage
- 4 c. water
- 2 celery bunch
- 2 small onion
- 4 carrots
- 1 t. of each:
- Ground mustard
- Ground coriander
- Ground marjoram
- Black pepper
- Salt
- Ground thyme

Directions:

1. Dice the carrots, onions, and celery and toss them into the cooker.
2. Pour in the water.
3. Combine the spices, rub the beef, and arrange in the cooker.
4. Secure the lid and cook on low for seven hours.
5. Remove the top layer of cabbage.
6. Wash and cut it into quarters it until ready to cook.
7. When the beef is done, add the cabbage, and cook for one hour on the low setting.
8. Serve and enjoy.

Kale And Chicken Broth Soup

Ingredients:

- 2 large chicken breast, cut into small strips
- 2 cups chopped fresh kale
- 6 garlic cloves, finely chopped
- 4 tbsp grated fresh ginger
- 6 cups chicken stock

Directions:

1. Drizzle some olive oil into the Crock Pot.
2. Add the garlic, ginger, stock, chicken breast, kale, salt, and pepper to the pot, stir to combine.
3. Place the lid onto the pot and set the temperature to HIGH.
4. Cook for 4 hours.

5. Serve this soup while steaming hot!.

Herbed Green Beans

Ingredients:

- 2 tablespoon of basil, diced
- 2 tablespoon of dill, diced
- A pinch of salt and black pepper
- 1 cup of almonds, diced
- 1 teaspoon of chili powder
- 2 lb. green beans, trimmed and halved
- 2 and 1 cups of chicken stock
- 2 tablespoon of rosemary, diced

Directions:

1. Start by throwing all the Ingredients: into the Crockpot.
2. Cover its lid and cook for 2 hours on Low setting.
3. Once done, remove its lid of the crockpot carefully.
4. Mix well and garnish as desired.
5. Serve warm.

Stuffed Parmesan Meatballs

Ingredients:

- 2 pinch of fresh parsley
- 2 tablespoon / 24gof Sukrin coconut flower
- 2 tablespoon / 24gof provolone cheese
- 2 tablespoon / 24gof walnuts, chopped
- 2 tablespoon / 24gof tomato paste
- 2 pinch of salt
- 2 small fresh egg
- 2 tablespoon / 24gof Parmesan cheese
- 2 tablespoons / 30 gr of ghee
- 2 tablespoon / 24gof coconut oil
- 2 pinch of salt

Directions:

1. Pour in a bowl the meat, egg, parmesan cheese, salt, ghee, parsley and flour.
2. Mix everything trying to get a mixture that is not too soft or too hard.
3. It must be easy to mold it by hand
4. Take 1/2 of the mixture, about 65g, and stuff in its center the provolone and chopped walnuts.
5. Close it to get a ball.
6. Repeat the operation until the stuffing is finished
7. Once you have the meatballs, put them in the Slow Cooker greased with non-sticking spray, and cover with the onion and tomato paste with a spoon
8. Let it cook for 4 and a half hours on HIGH temperature and then half an hour on LOW mode.
9. At half-cooking, turn the meatballs upside down

Okra Sauté

Ingredients:

- 2 teaspoon turmeric powder
- 2 tablespoon curry paste
- 2 tablespoons sour cream
- 1 cup heavy cream
- 2 -pound okra, chopped
- 2 chili pepper, minced
- 2 teaspoon coriander, ground

Directions:

1. In the slow cooker, mix the okra with the chili pepper and the other ingredients.
2. Close the lid and cook for 4 hours on Low.

Beet And Goat Cheese

Ingredients:

- 2 tablespoons of swerves
- 2 -pint mixed cherry tomatoes, halved
- 2-ounce pecans
- Salt and black pepper- to taste
- 2 tablespoon of olive oil
- 4-ounce goat cheese, crumbled
- 2 tablespoon of balsamic vinegar
- 2 red onion, sliced

Directions:

1. Start by throwing all the Ingredients: into your Crockpot except cheese.
2. Cover its lid and cook for 4 hours on Low setting.
3. Once done, remove its lid and give it a stir.
4. Garnish with goat cheese.
5. Serve warm.

Easy And Delicious Chicken Stew

Ingredients:

- 2 red onion, diced
- 2 garlic cloves, minced
- 2 teaspoon dry oregano
- 2 teaspoon dry thyme
- 2 teaspoon dried rosemary
- 2 cup cooking cream
- Salt and pepper to taste
- 2.2 pounds chicken thighs, de-boned and cubed
- 2 cup chicken broth + 2 cup hot water
- 4 diced celery sticks 2 cups fresh spinach

Directions:

1. Add all the ingredients to the crock-pot.
2. Cover, cook on low for 6-6- ½ hours.

Chicken And Olives Stew

Ingredients:

- 2 red bell pepper, chopped
- 2 teaspoon basil, dried
- 2 teaspoon sweet paprika
- 1 cup black olives, sliced
- 2 -pound chicken breast, skinless, boneless
- 2 tablespoon keto tomato sauce
- 1 cup of coconut milk

Directions:

1. In the slow cooker, mix the chicken with the coconut milk and the other ingredients.
2. Close the lid and cook the chicken for 6 hours on High.
3. Divide into bowls and serve

Beef And Onion Stew

Ingredients:

- 6 garlic cloves, crushed
- 2 beef stock cube
- 2 tsp dried mixed herbs
- 2 lb boneless stewing beef, cut into cubes
- 2 onions, roughly chopped

Directions:

1. Drizzle the Crock Pot with olive oil.
2. Brown the beef in an oiled fry pan or skillet for about 2 minutes to seal.
3. Place the beef, onions, garlic, stock cube, salt, pepper, herbs, and 4 cups of water to the pot.
4. Place the lid onto the pot.
5. Set the temperature to LOW.
6. Cook for 25 hours.

7. Remove the lid, stir the stew, and serve while hot, with a side of greens and mashed cauliflower.

Wine Glazed Mushrooms

Ingredients:

- 1/2 cup of white wine
- Salt to taste
- Black pepper to taste
- 6 garlic cloves, minced
- 2 lbs. fresh mushrooms, sliced
- 1/2 cup of balsamic vinegar

Directions:

1. Start by throwing all the Ingredients: into your Crockpot.
2. Cover its lid and cook for 4 hours on Low setting.
3. Once done, remove its lid and give it a stir.
4. Garnish as desired.
5. Serve warm.

Pesto Peppers

Ingredients:

- 1/2 teaspoon of Red pepper flakes, crushed
- Salt and black pepper- to taste
- Handful parsley, chopped
- 1 cup of vegetable stock
- 6 tablespoon of Jarred basil pesto
- 2 tablespoon of Lemon juice
- 2 tablespoon of Olive oil
- 2 lb. zucchini, sliced

Directions:

1. Start by throwing all the Ingredients: into your Crockpot.
2. Cover its lid and cook for 4 hours on Low setting.
3. Once done, remove its lid and give it a stir.
4. Garnish as desired.

5. Serve warm.

Garlicky Shrimp

Ingredients:

- Salt and pepper, to taste
- 5 lb. jumbo shrimp, shelled and deveined
- 1 cup olive oil
- 6 cloves of garlic, minced

Directions:

1. Place all ingredients in the crock pot and stir well.
2. Close the lid and cook on high for 2 hours.
3. Garnish with chopped fresh parsley if desired.

Coconut Okra

Ingredients:

- 1 teaspoon salt
- 1 teaspoon turmeric powder
- ¾ teaspoon ground nutmeg
- 2 -pound okra, trimmed
- 1/2 cup coconut cream
- 1/2 cup butter

Directions:

1. In the slow cooker, mix the okra with cream, butter and the other ingredients.
2. Cook okra for 4 hours on High.

Toscana Soup

Ingredients:

- Chopped kale   5 cups
- Cauliflower   1 head, diced florets
- Salt   1 tsp.
- Crushed red pepper flakes   1/2 tsp.
- Heavy cream   1/2 cup
- Pepper   1 tsp.
- Olive oil   2 tbsp.
- Onion   1/2 cup, diced
- Chicken stock   2 8 oz.
- Garlic   cloves, minced

Directions:

1. In a pan, brown the sausage.
2. Transfer the sausage to the Crock-Pot and discard the grease.
3. Add the oil into the skillet and sauté the onions for 4 to 4 minutes.
4. Add to the Crock-Pot.

5. Except for the cream, add the rest of the ingredients to the Crock-Pot.
6. Mix and cook on low for 8 hours.
7. Add the cream when cooked.
8. Stir and serve hot.

Easy Lamb Hotpot

Ingredients:

- 5 large potatoes in 4 mm slices
- 2 large carrot in bitesize pieces
- 1/2 lb. diced lamb leg

Directions:

1. In a crock-pot, add a little oil plus the onion and carrot.
2. Cover and cook on a low for 6 minutes or until soft but not brown.
3. Change to high then add lamb.
4. Cook for 2-4 minutes until browned.
5. Add the lamb stock and a little salt and pepper.
6. Arrange the potato slices for them to overlap slightly.
7. Cover and cook for 4 hours on high.

Crockpot Pork With Picante Sauce

Ingredients:

- 2 jar picante sauce
- Salt and pepper to taste
- 4 cloves of garlic, chopped
- 2 package frozen vegetables

Directions:

1. Heat skillet over fresh flame and add the pork cubes and garlic.
2. Stir until all sides turn slightly brown.
3. Transfer into the crockpot and add the vegetables and picante sauce.
4. Season with salt and pepper to taste.
5. Close the lid and cook on low for 8 hours.

French Onion Soup

Ingredients:

- 2 teaspoon turmeric powder
- 1 teaspoon ground black pepper
- 8 oz Parmesan, grated
- 2 tablespoon butter
- 2 cup of water
- 4 spring onions, chopped
- 1 cup coconut milk
- 1 cup coconut cream
- 1 teaspoon minced garlic

Directions:

1. Melt butter and pour it in the slow cooker.
2. Add the onions and the other ingredients except the cheese.
3. Close the lid and cook soup for 2 hours on High.

4. After this, add grated cheese and stir well.
5. Cook the soup for 2 hours more on Low.

Bacon And Cauliflower Soup

Ingredients:

- Bacon 4 slices, cut into small pieces
- Chicken stock 2 cups
- Smoked paprika 1 tsp.
- Chili powder 1 tsp.
- Heavy cream ¾ cup
- Olive oil 2 tbsp.
- Salt and pepper to taste
- Paprika to taste
- Garlic 4 cloves, crushed
- Onion ¾, finely chopped

Directions:

1. Add olive oil into the Crock-Pot.
2. Add the garlic, cauliflower, onion, bacon, stock, paprika, chili, salt, and pepper to the pot. Stir to mix.

148

3. Cover with the lid and cook on high for 4 hours.
4. Open the lid and blend with a hand mixer.
5. Add the cream and mix.
6. Serve sprinkled with paprika.

White Chicken Chili Soup

Ingredients:

- 2 2 jalapeño pepper, minced
- 25 cloves garlic, smashed
- 2 tablespoon of chili powder
- 2 teaspoon of cumin
- 2 teaspoon of oregano
- 1 teaspoon of black pepper
- Serve with cilantro
- 2 onions, diced
- 4 cups of chicken broth
- 2 teaspoon of coriander powder
- 4 stalks celery, diced
- 2 tablespoon of salt

Directions:

1. Start by throwing all the Ingredients: into your Crockpot.
2. Mix well and cover the Crockpot with its lid.

3. Select the High settings for 4 hours.
4. Serve warm.

Butter, Cheese Brussels Sprouts

Ingredients:

- 2 tablespoons of butter, melted
- Salt and black pepper- to taste
- 4 tablespoons of parmesan, grated
- 2 lemon, juiced

Directions:

1. Start by throwing all the Ingredients: into your Crockpot.
2. Cover its lid and cook for 4 hours on Low setting.
3. Once done, remove its lid and give it a stir.
4. Garnish as desired.
5. Serve warm.

Slow Cooker Bread Pudding

Ingredients:

- 2 fresh egg white
- 2 whole fresh egg
- 5 cups almond milk
- 4 slices of pumpkin bread
- 2 tablespoons raisin
- 1 teaspoon cinnamon
- 5 teaspoon vanilla extract
- 1/2 cup swerve

Directions:

1. Slice the pumpkin bread into pieces.
2. Then mix all the rest of the fixing in the slow cooker.
3. Cook within 4 to 6 hours, then serve.

153

Tiramisu Bread Pudding

Ingredients:

- Cooking spray - 4 1/2 cups Keto bread
- 2 large egg, lightly beaten
- 6.4 ounces of almond milk, divided
- 1/3 tablespoons Kahlua 2 1/3 teaspoons instant espresso granules
- 2 tablespoons coconut sugar
- 2 .6-ounce water
- 1/3 teaspoons unsweetened cocoa
- 1/2 teaspoon vanilla extract
- 2 tablespoons mascarpone cheese

Directions:

1. Mix the water, coconut sugar, plus instant espresso granules in a saucepan.
2. Boil while occasionally stirring for 2 minute, remove, then mix in the Kahlua liqueur.

3. Whisk the eggs, then the almond milk in a large bowl.
4. Mix in the espresso mixture into it.
5. Put the Keto friendly bread into a greased casserole.
6. Cook it inside the slow cooker within 2 hours, low.
7. Mix vanilla, mascarpone cheese plus the remaining almond milk in a bowl.
8. Garnish with cocoa and serve.

Crock Pot Sugar-Free Dairy-Free Fudge

Ingredients:

- 1 tablespoon coconut milk
- 4 tablespoons sugar-free chocolate chips
- 1/2 teaspoons vanilla liquid stevia
- A dash of salt - Dash of pure vanilla extract

Directions:

1. Mix in coconut milk, stevia, vanilla, chocolate chips plus salt in a slow cooker.
2. Cook within 2 hours, then let it sit within 45 minutes.
3. Mix in within 6 minutes.
4. Put the batter in a casserole dish with parchment paper.
5. Chill, then serve.

Poppy Seed-Lemon Bread

Ingredients:

- 2 /8 tsp salt
- 2 tbsp vegetable oil
- 4 tbsp tofu
- 1/2 cup almond milk
- 1/3 cup plain Greek-style yogurt
- 1/2 cup lemon juice
- 1/3 tsp shredded lemon peel
- 1/2 tsp vanilla
- 1 cups almond flour
- 1/2 tbsp baking powder
- 2 tbsp poppy seeds
- 2 fresh egg
- 1/2 cup coconut sugar

Directions:

1. Grease the slow cooker using a non-stick cooking spray.

2. Mix the poppy seeds, flour, salt, and baking powder in a bowl, then put it aside.
3. Mix the tofu puree, sugar, oil, milk, yogurt, lemon juice, lemon peel, and vanilla in a fresh bowl.
4. Put the sugar batter to the flour batter, then mix.
5. Transfer it in the slow cooker, then cook on high for 2 and 45 minutes to 2 hours, or until set.
6. Leave for 2 0-35 minutes to cool., then serve.

Spicy Mushroom Soup

Ingredients:

- 2 bunch fresh cilantro, diced
- 2 tablespoon of soy sauce
- 2 tablespoon of olive oil
- 2 tablespoons of garlic, minced
- 2 tablespoon of chili powder
- 1 teaspoon of ground ginger
- 2 red chili, sliced
- 25 oz. ramen noodles
- 6 cups of chicken broth stock
- 2 cup of mushrooms, sliced

Directions:

1. Start by throwing all the Ingredients: except cilantro and red chili into your Crockpot.
2. Mix well and cover the Crockpot with its lid.

159

3. Select the Low settings for 6 hours.
4. Garnish with red chili and cilantro.
5. Serve warm.

Kale Chowder

Ingredients:

- 1 teaspoon curry powder
- 1/2 cup spring onions, chopped
- 2 tablespoon chives, chopped
- 1 cup chicken stock
- 2 teaspoon salt
- 2 cup organic coconut milk
- 8 oz kale, chopped
- 2 teaspoon ground black pepper
- 2 tablespoon coconut cream

Directions:

1. In the slow cooker, mix the kale with coconut milk, cream and the other ingredients, close the lid and cook on High for 4 hours.
2. Blend using an immersion blender, divide into bowls and serve.

161

Coconut Chicken

Ingredients:

- Coconut milk, unsweetened, full-fat   2 cup
- Salt ¾ teaspoon
- Ground black pepper   1 teaspoon
- Chicken breast, cubed   2 pound
- Chicken broth   2 cup
- Stalks of lemongrass   6

Directions:

1. Switch on the instant pot, add celery, then top with chicken, add lemongrass and pour in chicken broth.
2. Shut the instant pot with its lid in the sealed position, then press the 'manual' button, press '+/-' to set the cooking time to 22 minutes and cook at high-pressure setting; when the pressure

builds in the pot, the cooking timer will start.

3. When the instant pot buzzes, press the 'keep warm' button, do a quick pressure release and open the lid.

4. Remove and discard lemongrass, season with salt and black pepper, then pour in coconut milk and stir until combined.

5. Serve coconut chicken with cauliflower rice.

Spicy Pork

Ingredients:

- 2 tablespoon sea salt
- 1 teaspoon ground black pepper
- 5 tablespoon paprika, divided
- 1 tablespoon dried oregano
- 1 tablespoon ground cumin
- 2 limes, juiced
- 2 tablespoons avocado oil
- 1 of jalapeno, deseeded and cored, chopped
- 6 ounce crushed tomatoes
- 1/2 cup chopped green onion
- 4 clove of garlic, peeled and sliced in half

Directions:

1. Place pork in a 6-quart slow cooker, season with salt, black pepper, paprika, oregano, and cumin until seasoned well.
2. Then add remaining ingredients and stir until combined.
3. Plug in the slow cooker, shut it with the lid and cook for 8 to 25 hours at low heat setting or 4 to 6 hours at high heat setting until very tender.
4. Serve straightaway.

Tomato Soup

Ingredients:

- 2 teaspoon of dried basil, crushed
- Black pepper, to taste
- 2 cups of vegetable broth
- 2 tablespoons of Erythritol
- 1 tablespoon of balsamic vinegar
- 1/2 cup of fresh basil, diced
- 2 small onion, diced
- 2 garlic clove, minced
- 5 lb. tomatoes, diced
- 2 tablespoon of sugar-free tomato sauce
- 2 teaspoon of parsley, dried, crushed

Directions:

1. Start by throwing all the Ingredients: into your Crockpot.
2. Cover its lid and cook for 2 hours on High setting.

166

3. Once done, remove its lid and give it a stir.
4. Garnish as desired.
5. Serve warm.

Crock Pot Jalapeno Chicken Chili

Ingredients:

- 2 teaspoons smoked paprika
- 2 teaspoons chili powder
- 2 teaspoons dried oregano
- 2 teaspoons sea salt
- 2 teaspoon ground cumin
- 1/2 teaspoon red pepper flakes
- 2 can petite diced tomatoes
- Chopped scallions for garnish
- 8 ounces of avocado, diced
- 4 ounces goat cheese
- 4 garlic cloves, minced
- 2 red bell pepper, diced
- 2 jalapenos, seeds removed
- 2 large sweet potato,
- 2 lb. lean ground chicken
- 2 lb. lean ground beef

Directions:

1. Place all the ingredients into your Crock Pot, except for goat cheese, scallions, and avocado.
2. Cover and cook on LOW for 8 hours.
3. When done, break up meat using wooden spoon, then add in half of goat cheese.
4. Serve garnished with scallions, avocado and remaining goat cheese.

Butter Green Peas

Ingredients:

- 2 tablespoon olive oil
- ¾ teaspoon salt
- 2 teaspoon paprika
- 2 teaspoon garam masala
- 1 cup chicken stock
- 2 cup green peas
- 2 teaspoon minced garlic
- 2 tablespoon butter, softened
- 1 teaspoon cayenne pepper

Directions:

1. In the slow cooker, mix the peas with butter, garlic and the other ingredients,
2. Close the lid and cook for 4 hours on High.

Dill Mixed Fennel Bulbs

Ingredients:

- 2 tablespoon of dill, diced
- 2 tablespoon of parsley, chopped
- 1/2 cup of chicken stock
- A pinch of salt and black pepper

Directions:

1. Start by throwing all the Ingredients: into the Crockpot.
2. Cover its lid and cook for 4 hours on Low setting.
3. Once done, remove its lid of the crockpot carefully.
4. Mix well and garnish as desired.
5. Serve warm.

Beef Mince, Tomato, And Sausage Chili

Ingredients:

- 2 beef stock cube
- 2 tsp smoked paprika
- 2 tsp dried chili flakes
- 4 sausages, cut into pieces
- 2 lb minced beef
- 2 onion, finely chopped
- 4 garlic cloves, crushed
- 4 tomatoes, chopped

Directions:

1. Drizzle some olive oil into the Crock Pot.
2. Add the minced beef, onion, garlic, tinned tomatoes, stock cube, paprika, chili, sausages, salt, pepper, and one cup of water to the pot, stir to combine.
3. Place the lid onto the pot and set the temperature to LOW.

4. Cook for 8 hours.
5. Remove the lid, stir the chili, and serve while hot!

Cabbage Stew

Ingredients:

- 2 teaspoon ground black pepper
- 1 cup spring onions, chopped
- 2 teaspoon chili flakes
- ¾ tablespoon keto tomatoes sauce
- 1/2 cup water
- 2 tablespoon dill, chopped
- 2 -pound white cabbage, shredded
- 2 cup cherry tomatoes, halved
- 5 cup ground pork
- 2 teaspoon salt

Directions:

1. In the slow cooker, mix the cabbage with the tomatoes and the other ingredients.

2. Close the lid and cook the stew for 8
   hours on Low.
3. Divide into bowls and serve.

Creamy Coconut Cauliflower

Ingredients:

- A pinch of salt and black pepper
- 2 tablespoons of balsamic vinegar
- 2 cup of coconut cream
- 2 cup of red onion, diced
- 1/2 cup of chicken stock

Directions:

1. Start by throwing all the Ingredients: into the Crockpot.
2. Cover its lid and cook for 4 hours on Low setting.
3. Once done, remove its lid of the crockpot carefully.
4. Mix well and garnish as desired.
5. Serve warm.

Lettuce Boats With Beef Mince, Parmesan, And Pumpkin Seeds

Ingredients:

- 1 cup grated parmesan cheese
- 1/2 cup pumpkin seeds
- 1 cos lettuce leaves
- 2 lb beef mince
- 2 garlic cloves, crushed

Directions:

1. Drizzle some olive oil into the Crock Pot.
2. Add the beef mince, garlic, parmesan, salt, and pepper and stir to combine.
3. Add the lid to the pot and set the temperature to HIGH.
4. Cook for 2 hours or until the beef has cooked through and the parmesan has melted.

5. Fill each lettuce cup with a large spoonful of warm mince mixture and sprinkle the pumpkin seeds over the top.
6. Serve on a platter with a drizzle of olive oil and a sprinkling of sea salt and freshly cracked pepper.

CPSIA information can be obtained
at www.ICGtesting.com
Printed in the USA
LVHW050452100221
678895LV00007B/1097

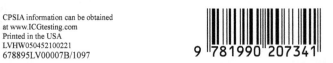